Anti-inflammatory diet for beginners

A 21-Day Anti-Inflammatory Meal Plan with 100+ Easy Recipes to Support Joint Health, Improve Digestion, and Boost Energy Naturally

Abigail Douglas

Table of Contents

Disclaimer

This book is for educational and informational purposes only and is not intended as medical advice. Always consult with a qualified healthcare professional before making any dietary, lifestyle, or supplement changes, especially if you have existing health conditions or are taking medications. The author and publisher disclaim responsibility for any adverse effects that may result from the use of information presented herein.

Preface

Inflammation has become the silent burden of modern life. For millions of people, it shows up as aching joints, stubborn belly fat, brain fog, digestive distress, fatigue, or the nagging feeling that something inside is always "off." You may not see it on the surface, but chronic inflammation quietly chips away at energy, focus, and long-term health.

When I began writing Anti-Inflammatory Diet for Beginners, my goal was simple: to create a guide that strips away the overwhelm and makes healing through food not only possible but enjoyable. There are countless diet books that promise quick fixes, but very few that meet you where you are—at the kitchen table, in the grocery aisle, or in that moment of decision when cravings hit. This book is about real life.

The truth is, your body has incredible power to heal when you give it the right tools. Every meal you eat can either fuel inflammation or fight it. That's why this book combines a **21-Day Anti-Inflammatory Meal Plan, 100+ easy recipes**, and **simple grocery lists** to give you a clear, practical roadmap to reducing pain, restoring gut health, supporting weight loss, and boosting energy naturally.

You'll find breakfasts that energize instead of crash, lunches that travel well, comforting one-pan dinners, smart snacks that truly satisfy, and guilt-free desserts you can enjoy without regret. Each recipe is built on whole, healing foods—leafy greens, berries, salmon, quinoa, turmeric, ginger, olive oil—that have been proven to calm inflammation and support long-term health.

But more than a collection of recipes, this is a reset for your entire lifestyle. In these pages, you'll learn how to:

- Remove inflammatory triggers like sugar, refined carbs, and processed oils.
- Heal your gut with probiotics, fiber-rich foods, and plant diversity.
- Support joint health, balance hormones, and strengthen your immune system.
- Use simple meal prep hacks to make healthy eating fit into busy days.
- Build lasting habits with flexible frameworks like the 80/20 approach—so you never feel restricted.

This book is for anyone who's tired of quick fixes and ready for a sustainable, healing path forward. Whether your goal is **to lose weight, reduce inflammation, heal your gut, boost energy, or simply eat cleaner**, you'll find a step-by-step plan here that works for beginners and beyond.

The recipes are designed to be realistic and accessible—5 ingredients, 20 minutes, affordable grocery staples—so you don't feel chained to the kitchen or your wallet. You'll also find shopping lists, printable meal plans, and lifestyle strategies that make it easier than ever to take the guesswork out of eating well.

If you've struggled with fatigue, inflammation, or diets that don't last, let this book be your fresh start. Within just a few weeks, you'll notice the difference: less bloating, lighter joints, clearer focus, and a renewed sense of vitality.

Your journey begins now, not with restriction but with empowerment. With each recipe, each meal, and each day of the plan, you'll be fueling healing from the inside out.

Let's step into a new chapter together—one where food is medicine, inflammation is no longer in control, and every bite moves you closer to the vibrant, pain-free life you deserve.

Introduction

Why Inflammation Is the Silent Enemy

You can't see it, and you may not even know it's there—but inflammation quietly shapes the way your body feels every single day. It's the silent enemy behind stiff joints when you wake up, the fatigue that lingers no matter how much you sleep, the bloating or gut discomfort you can't explain, and even the brain fog that makes it hard to think clearly.

Not all inflammation is bad. In fact, acute inflammation is your body's natural defense mechanism—how it heals a cut, repairs a sprained ankle, or fights off an infection. That type of inflammation is short-lived and essential for survival. The problem arises when inflammation becomes chronic. Instead of switching off once the body has healed, it lingers. Slowly, quietly, it chips away at your energy, mobility, and long-term health.

Chronic inflammation has been linked to some of the most common struggles of modern life: joint pain, digestive issues, fatigue, skin flare-ups, and even weight gain that seems impossible to lose. Left unchecked, it can contribute to serious conditions like heart disease, type 2 diabetes, and autoimmune disorders. The frustrating part? You may not even realize it's happening until the symptoms are impossible to ignore.

Here's the good news: food is one of the most powerful tools you have to fight back. Every bite you take either fuels inflammation or helps calm it. Sugary drinks, fried foods, and refined carbs can stoke the fire, while omega-3-rich salmon, antioxidant-packed berries, and spices like turmeric and ginger act like natural fire extinguishers. You don't need complicated supplements or extreme diets— the right ingredients, eaten consistently, can transform how you feel.

That's why this book exists: to give you a simple, structured, and beginner-friendly path to reclaim your health through food. Inside, you'll find a clear 21-day meal plan designed to lower inflammation, balance digestion, and restore energy. You'll also discover over 100 easy, delicious recipes that prove healthy eating doesn't mean boring or restrictive meals.

Whether you're tired of joint stiffness, want to heal your gut, or simply crave more energy for everyday life, this guide will help you take back control—one meal, one day, one small choice at a time.

This isn't a fad diet. It's a reset—a way to quiet the inflammation that's been holding you back and to rebuild your foundation of health naturally. And the best part? You don't have to do it alone. This book will walk with you, step by step, until anti-inflammatory eating becomes second nature.

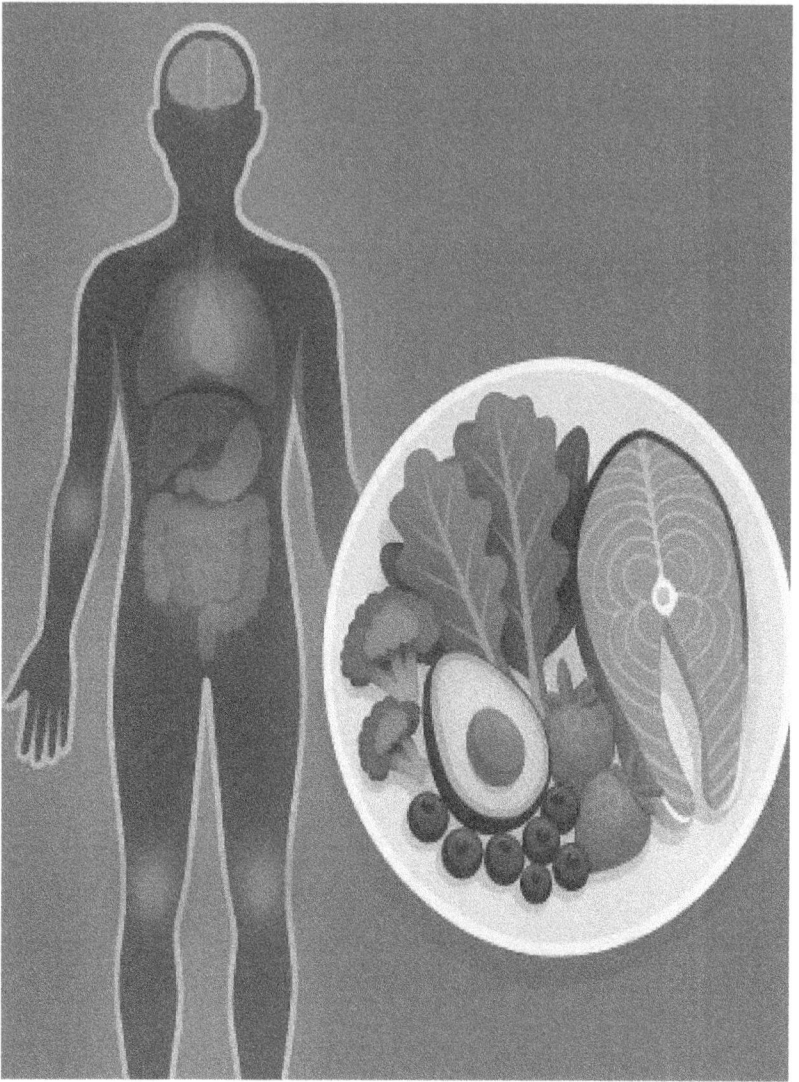

PART I – THE BEGINNER'S BLUEPRINT

Chapter 1

Understanding Inflammation and Healing Through Food

If you've ever twisted an ankle or cut your finger, you've seen inflammation at work. The swelling, redness, and heat that follow are your body's natural way of protecting and repairing itself. In this short-term form—what doctors call **acute inflammation**—it's a powerful ally. Without it, wounds wouldn't heal and infections could spread unchecked.

But inflammation also has a darker side. When it doesn't switch off as it should, it lingers in the background, quietly damaging tissues and organs over time. This is known as **chronic inflammation**, and it's the type most of us struggle with without realizing it. Unlike a swollen ankle, chronic inflammation doesn't always make itself obvious.

22

Instead, it shows up as stiff joints in the morning, unexplained fatigue, frequent bloating, skin flare-ups, brain fog, or even weight gain that feels stubborn no matter how hard you try. Left unaddressed, it has been linked to conditions such as arthritis, heart disease, type 2 diabetes, autoimmune disorders, and even certain cancers.

The Difference Between Good and Bad Inflammation

- **Good (Acute) Inflammation:**

This is short-lived and purposeful. If you scrape your knee, white blood cells rush to the site to fight infection and begin the healing process. Within a few days, as the injury heals, the inflammation fades away.

- **Bad (Chronic) Inflammation:**

Here, the body's defense system becomes overactive,

sometimes due to poor diet, chronic stress, lack of sleep, or environmental toxins. Instead of protecting you, it starts to harm you, fueling a low-grade fire inside your body that can persist for years.

Think of it like this: a campfire is helpful when controlled—it warms you, cooks your food, lights your night. But when sparks leap out of the pit and spread across dry grass, that same fire can become destructive. Chronic inflammation is those sparks gone wild, damaging systems you rely on every day.

Common Triggers of Inflammation

Modern diets are full of foods that act like gasoline on this fire. While they may be convenient or tasty in the moment, they set the stage for fatigue, gut issues, and long-term health problems:

- **Sugar:** Refined sugar spikes blood sugar and insulin, which encourages inflammatory processes in the body.

- **Refined Carbohydrates:** White bread, pasta, pastries, and other highly processed carbs break down quickly into sugar, producing the same effect as sweets.

- **Processed Oils:** Industrial seed oils like soybean, corn, and canola are often high in omega-6 fatty acids, which, in excess, can throw off your body's balance and fuel inflammation.

- **Alcohol:** Occasional moderate use may be fine for some, but frequent or heavy drinking stresses the liver and promotes gut inflammation.

- **Ultra-Processed Foods:** Packaged snacks, fast food, and ready meals often combine all of the above—sugar, refined carbs, and unhealthy oils— making them some of the worst offenders.

These are the culprits many of us consume daily without realizing the slow, cumulative toll they take.

Foods That Fight Inflammation

The beauty of your body is that it responds quickly when you give it the right fuel. Just as certain foods stoke inflammation, others act like natural fire extinguishers. Incorporating them into your daily meals can reduce symptoms, support healing, and protect against disease.

- **Fatty Fish:** Salmon, mackerel, and sardines are rich in omega-3 fatty acids, which directly combat inflammatory pathways.
- **Berries:** Blueberries, strawberries, and raspberries contain antioxidants called anthocyanins, which reduce oxidative stress.

- **Olive Oil:** Especially extra-virgin, it's loaded with monounsaturated fats and anti-inflammatory compounds like oleocanthal.
- **Turmeric:** This golden spice contains curcumin, a powerful natural anti-inflammatory often compared to over-the-counter pain relievers.
- **Ginger:** Known for soothing digestion, it also helps reduce inflammatory markers in the body.
- **Leafy Greens:** Spinach, kale, and Swiss chard are nutrient powerhouses rich in vitamins, minerals, and phytonutrients.

These foods don't just fight inflammation in isolation; together, they create a protective web that supports gut health, brain clarity, and long-term vitality.

The Science in Plain English

When you hear terms like antioxidants, omega-3s, or

phytonutrients, it's easy to feel overwhelmed—as if you're reading a textbook. But here's what they really mean in everyday language:

- **Antioxidants:** Think of them as bodyguards for your cells. Every day, natural processes and environmental toxins create unstable molecules called free radicals. Left unchecked, they damage your cells, fueling inflammation. Antioxidants from foods like berries, dark chocolate, and leafy greens neutralize these free radicals, protecting your body from harm.

- **Omega-3s:** These are healthy fats found in fatty fish, chia seeds, and flaxseeds. Omega-3s are like the peacekeepers of your body, calming inflammatory pathways and balancing out the effects of omega-6s (which tend to be overconsumed in modern diets).

- **Phytonutrients:** These are natural plant compounds that act like microscopic healers. Found in colorful fruits, vegetables, herbs, and spices, they help regulate your immune system, reduce oxidative stress, and support the gut-brain connection. Each color—red tomatoes, green spinach, orange turmeric—offers its own unique set of benefits.

When you fill your plate with foods rich in these compounds, you're giving your body the tools it needs to fight inflammation naturally, gently, and effectively.

Bringing It All Together

Understanding inflammation doesn't have to be complicated. The message is simple: avoid the foods that fuel the fire, and embrace those that help put it out. Small, consistent changes—like swapping sugary cereal for a berry smoothie, or using olive oil instead of vegetable oil—make a real difference.

The best part? Your body responds quickly. Many people notice reduced bloating, less stiffness, and more stable energy levels within just a couple of weeks of eating this way.

And that's exactly what this book is here to guide you through—a practical, step-by-step reset. In the next chapter, we'll get hands-on: setting up your pantry, planning your grocery list, and preparing for the 21-day journey that will help you feel lighter, clearer, and more energized.

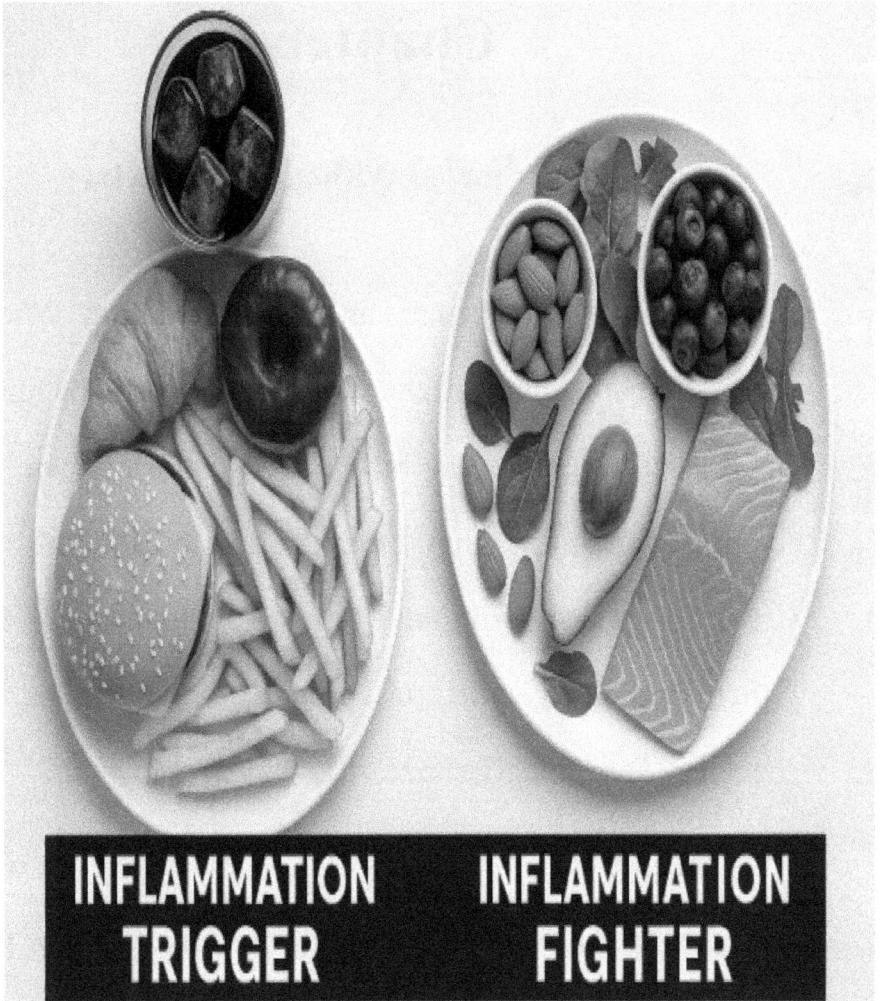

INFLAMMATION TRIGGER INFLAMMATION FIGHTER

Chapter 2

Getting Started Without Overwhelm

Making a lifestyle change can feel intimidating. When it comes to eating anti-inflammatory foods, many beginners imagine a long grocery bill, hours in the kitchen, and complicated recipes they'll never stick to. But here's the truth: this reset doesn't have to be overwhelming. In fact, when you set yourself up properly from the start, it becomes surprisingly simple—and even enjoyable.

This chapter is about making those first steps easy, clear, and doable. Think of it as creating the foundation of your new kitchen: you're not tearing your life apart, just reshaping your space so that the healthy choice becomes the convenient choice.

Pantry Reset: What to Toss and What to Stock Up On

Your pantry is the heartbeat of your diet. If it's filled with processed snacks and sugary temptations, every mealtime decision becomes harder. If, instead, it's stocked with nourishing staples, healthy eating becomes effortless.

What to Toss (or gradually phase out):

- **Sugary foods:** candy, cookies, sweetened cereals, soda.
- **Refined carbs:** white bread, pasta, pastries.
- **Processed oils:** soybean, corn, vegetable, or canola oil.
- **Ultra-processed snacks:** chips, crackers, microwave dinners.
- **Alcohol excess:** keep for special occasions, not daily habit.

What to Stock Up On:

- **Whole grains:** quinoa, brown rice, oats.

- **Healthy fats:** extra-virgin olive oil, avocado oil, nuts, seeds.

- **Lean proteins:** salmon, chicken, lentils, beans.

- **Herbs and spices:** turmeric, ginger, cinnamon, garlic.

- **Fresh and frozen vegetables:** spinach, kale, broccoli, mixed greens.

- **Fruits:** berries, apples, citrus, bananas for quick energy.

Tip: *Don't feel pressured to throw everything out at once. As you use up the old, replace it with better choices. The goal is progress, not perfection.*

Grocery Shopping Made Easy

Many people think healthy eating means expensive health-store trips, but the anti-inflammatory diet can be as simple as shopping smart at your local market.

- **Fresh Produce:** Buy seasonal fruits and vegetables—they're cheaper, fresher, and tastier.

- **Frozen Options:** Frozen spinach, berries, and broccoli are just as nutritious as fresh and often more affordable. Keep them in your freezer for quick meals.

- **Canned Staples:** Chickpeas, black beans, tuna, and salmon (choose BPA-free cans in water or olive oil) can make quick, budget-friendly meals.

- **Bulk Buying:** Stock up on nuts, oats, brown rice, and quinoa in larger quantities to save money long-term.

Make a shopping list before you go—it helps you stay focused, save money, and resist impulse buys.

Budget-Friendly Tips

Eating well doesn't mean overspending. Here's how to make your anti-inflammatory reset sustainable:

1. **Meal Prepping:** Cook once, eat multiple times. For example, roast a tray of vegetables and use them in salads, wraps, and grain bowls throughout the week.

2. **Seasonal Buying:** Strawberries are cheaper in summer, squash is cheaper in fall. Build your menu around what's in season to cut costs.

3. **Plan Leftovers:** Make extra portions of soups or stews and freeze them for quick meals later.

4. **Cook Simple Meals:** You don't need a five-course menu. A piece of salmon, a serving of quinoa, and steamed broccoli is quick, affordable, and nutrient-packed.

Portion Control and Balance

The anti-inflammatory diet isn't about strict calorie counting—it's about balance and nourishment. To feel satisfied and energized, each meal should have:

- **Protein:** Supports muscles, repairs tissues, keeps you full.

- **Carbohydrates (the right kind):** Whole grains, legumes, or root vegetables for steady energy.

- **Healthy Fats:** Olive oil, avocado, nuts, or fatty fish to calm inflammation and support brain health.

- **Fiber & Micronutrients:** Vegetables and fruits for gut health, digestion, and natural detox.

A simple way to balance your plate:

- Fill **half your plate** with vegetables and fruits.
- Fill **one-quarter** with lean protein.
- Fill **one-quarter** with whole grains or starchy vegetables.

- Add a small serving of healthy fats (a drizzle of olive oil, a few slices of avocado, a handful of nuts).

Think of portion balance not as a rigid rule but as a guide to keep your meals satisfying and healing.

The Takeaway

Getting started doesn't have to be overwhelming. By cleaning out your pantry, shopping smart, cooking simple meals, and balancing your plate, you're building a foundation for a lifestyle that supports energy, healing, and long-term health.

In the next chapter, we'll bring it all together in your **21-day anti-inflammatory reset plan**—a practical, step-by-step roadmap to calm inflammation, heal your gut, and boost your energy naturally.

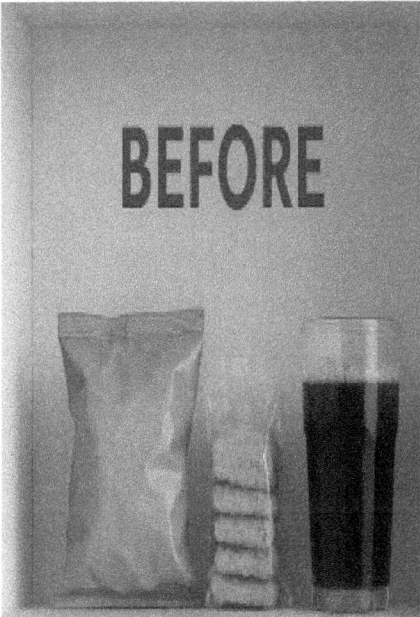
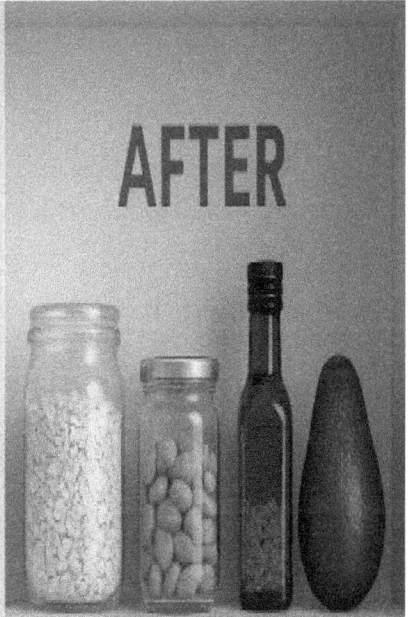
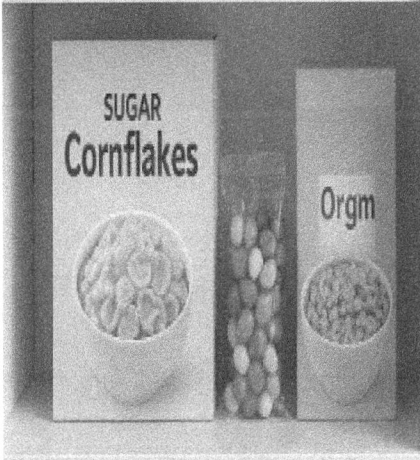
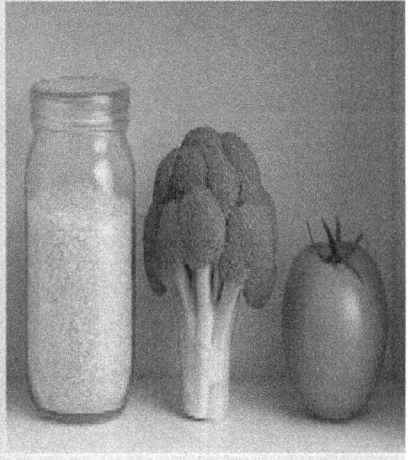

Chapter 3

The 21-Day Anti-Inflammatory Reset

When you're trying to change your health, the hardest part is often getting started. That's why this plan is built around **21 days**—a timeframe long enough to deliver noticeable results, but short enough to feel realistic and achievable. Think of it as a reset button for your body, helping you calm inflammation, restore balance, and rebuild energy without feeling overwhelmed.

Why 21 Days Works

There's a reason so many lifestyle programs use the 21-day model: it strikes the sweet spot between quick wins and lasting change.

- **It's long enough to see results.** Many people notice reduced bloating, improved digestion, and lighter joints in as little as 10–14 days. By 21 days, these changes become more consistent and visible.

- **It's short enough to commit to.** A month or more can feel daunting, but three weeks is manageable—even with a busy schedule.

- **It helps form habits.** Research suggests it takes about three weeks of repetition to begin rewiring daily routines. By the end of this plan, you'll already have the rhythm of cooking, eating, and shopping anti-inflammatory built into your lifestyle.

Week 1: Calm the Fire

Your first week is about **removing inflammatory triggers** and giving your body a gentle reset.

- **Focus:** Cut back on sugar, refined carbs, processed oils, and excess alcohol.

41

- **What to Eat:** Simple, soothing meals with lean proteins, leafy greens, berries, and healthy fats.
- **Goal:** Reduce bloat, joint stiffness, and energy crashes by stopping the constant "sparks" of inflammation.
- **Sample Meals:**
  - **Breakfast:** Overnight oats with chia and blueberries.
  - **Lunch:** Quinoa salad with leafy greens, avocado, and salmon.
  - **Dinner:** Turmeric chicken soup with carrots and spinach.

By the end of week one, most people report less bloating, lighter digestion, and a more stable energy curve throughout the day.

Week 2: Heal the Gut

Now that the fire is cooling, it's time to **restore balance in your digestive system**. Your gut is home to trillions of bacteria, many of which play a vital role in inflammation. By feeding the good bacteria, you help your body regulate itself.

- **Focus:** Add diversity—fiber-rich vegetables, fermented foods, and gut-friendly herbs.
- **What to Eat:** Probiotic-rich foods like yogurt, kefir, miso, and sauerkraut; fiber-rich legumes and vegetables.
- **Goal:** Support digestion, reduce brain fog, and improve nutrient absorption.
- **Sample Meals:**
- **Breakfast:** Greek yogurt parfait with berries and walnuts.

- **Lunch:** Lentil and veggie soup with turmeric and ginger.
- **Dinner:** Grilled shrimp stir-fry with broccoli, bell peppers, and ginger-lime sauce.

By the end of week two, many people notice improved digestion, fewer sugar cravings, and better mental clarity.

Week 3: Boost Energy & Sustain Habits

The final week isn't about restriction—it's about building momentum. With inflammation reduced and digestion improved, you'll focus on energy, balance, and sustainability.

- **Focus:** Fine-tune your meals to maintain energy all day and practice habits you can carry forward.

- **What to Eat:** A balanced mix of protein, healthy fats, whole grains, and plenty of colorful vegetables.

- **Goal:** Lock in sustainable routines for long-term health.

- **Sample Meals:**

- **Breakfast:** Green power smoothie with spinach, chia, and almond butter.

- **Lunch:** Roasted veggie quinoa bowl with tahini dressing.

- **Dinner:** Baked salmon with sweet potato mash and garlic-roasted greens.

By the end of week three, most people feel lighter, clearer, and more energized—and they've built habits they can continue for months or years.

Tracking Your Progress

It's easy to miss progress when you're living it day to day, so tracking is key. Here are simple ways to measure your improvements:

- **Joint Relief:** Notice if your morning stiffness eases or if everyday movements feel smoother.

- **Digestion:** Track bloating, bathroom regularity, and comfort after meals.

- **Energy Levels:** Write down how you feel in the mornings and afternoons compared to before starting.

- **Mood & Focus:** Many people report reduced brain fog and steadier moods.

You don't need complicated charts—a simple notebook or notes app works fine. Just jot down observations every 2–3 days. By the end of 21 days, you'll have a clear picture of how much has shifted.

The Takeaway

The 21-Day Anti-Inflammatory Reset is more than a meal plan—it's a new rhythm for your body. By moving through these three focused weeks, you'll calm the fire, heal the gut, and rebuild your energy. But perhaps the biggest benefit is this: you'll realize that anti-inflammatory living is not a temporary diet, but a sustainable way to feel your best.

In the next section, we'll dive into the **week-by-week** meal plans, giving you everything you need—recipes, shopping lists, and prep tips—to make this reset as effortless as possible.

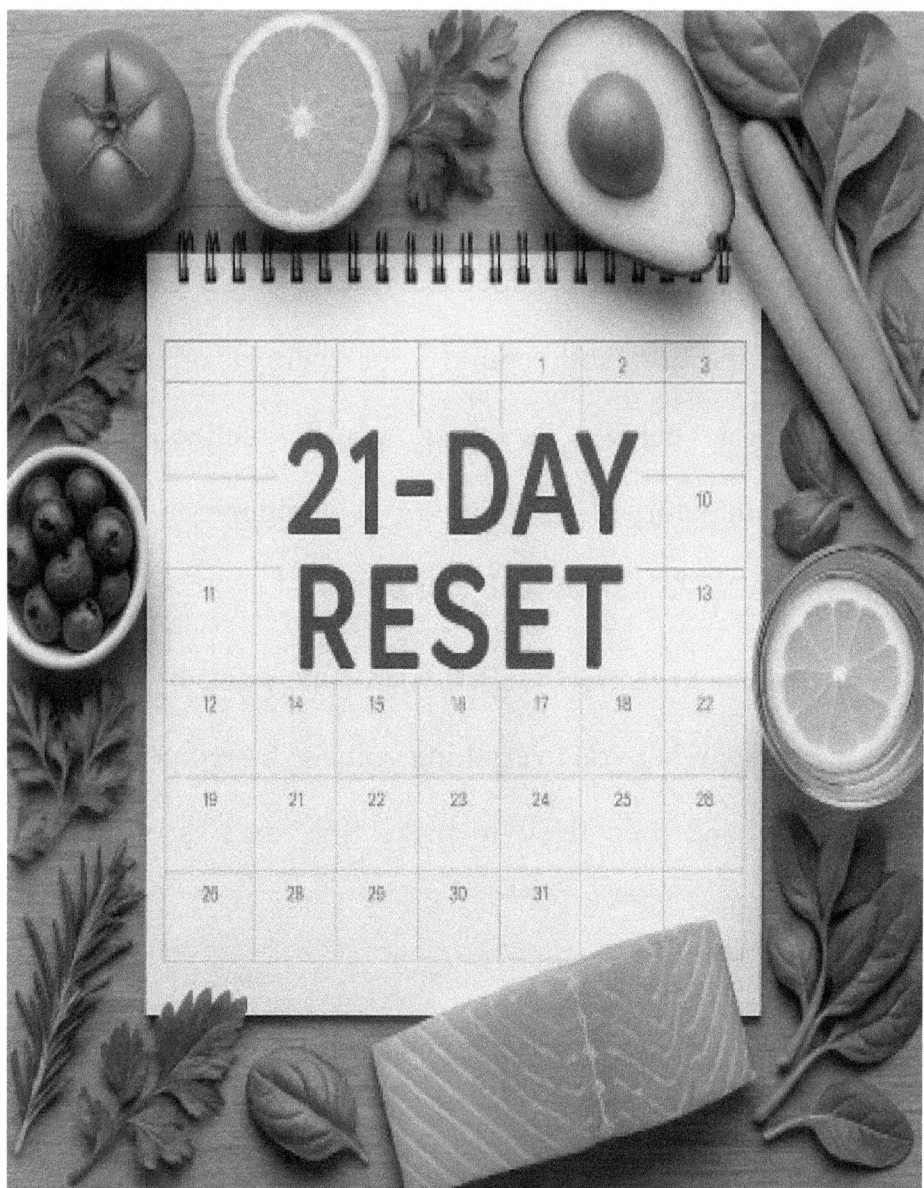

PART II – YOUR 21-DAY MEAL PLAN

Chapter 4

Week 1 - Calm the Fire

The first step in your 21-day anti-inflammatory reset is to cool the flames. In this week, you'll begin by **removing the most common inflammation triggers** and replacing them with simple, soothing meals that are easy to prepare and enjoyable to eat.

Think of this as giving your body a break from the constant sparks that fuel chronic inflammation—sugar, processed carbs, alcohol, and refined oils. By dialing these down, you'll give your system space to reset and begin to heal. The focus isn't perfection; it's awareness. Each choice you make is another step toward feeling lighter, clearer, and more energized.

Focus: Removing Triggers, Starting Simple

This week, you'll:

- Swap **sugary cereals or pastries** for breakfasts built on fiber, fruit, and healthy fats.
- Replace **fried and processed lunches** with bowls rich in lean proteins and vegetables.
- Cook **simple dinners** that fuel your body without leaving you sluggish.
- Keep **snacks wholesome** so you stay satisfied without the sugar crash.

By simplifying your meals, you'll notice how much easier it is to listen to your body's signals.

Your 7-Day Plan

Below is a sample structure for Week 1. Feel free to mix and match recipes, but try to stay within these meal

51

frameworks to give your body consistency.

Day 1

- **Breakfast:** Overnight oats with chia seeds, blueberries, and almond milk.

- **Lunch:** Quinoa salad with leafy greens, avocado, and grilled salmon.

- **Dinner:** Turmeric chicken soup with spinach, carrots, and garlic.

- **Snack:** A handful of almonds and an apple.

Day 2

- **Breakfast:** Greek yogurt with strawberries and flaxseed.

- **Lunch:** Lentil and vegetable stew with turmeric and ginger.

- **Dinner:** Grilled chicken breast with roasted sweet potatoes and broccoli.

- **Snack:** Carrot sticks with hummus.

Day 3

- **Breakfast:** Smoothie with spinach, banana, almond butter, and chia seeds.
- **Lunch:** Wild rice and roasted vegetable bowl with olive oil drizzle.
- **Dinner:** Baked salmon with garlic green beans and quinoa.
- **Snack:** Blueberries and a few walnuts.

Day 4

- **Breakfast:** Scrambled eggs with spinach and avocado slices.
- **Lunch:** Chickpea salad with cucumbers, tomatoes, and lemon-tahini dressing.
- **Dinner:** Turmeric chicken soup (double batch for leftovers).
- **Snack:** Sliced cucumber with guacamole.

Day 5

- **Breakfast:** Chia pudding made with almond milk, topped with raspberries.

- **Lunch:** Grilled shrimp with zucchini noodles and olive oil.

- **Dinner:** Quinoa and roasted vegetable stuffed peppers.

- **Snack:** Handful of pumpkin seeds and an orange.

Day 6

- **Breakfast:** Oatmeal topped with cinnamon, walnuts, and blueberries.

- **Lunch:** Turkey lettuce wraps with avocado and shredded carrots.

- **Dinner:** Baked cod with lemon, steamed asparagus, and wild rice.

- **Snack:** Greek yogurt with flaxseed.

Day 7

- **Breakfast:** Smoothie bowl with spinach, frozen mango, chia seeds, and coconut flakes.

- **Lunch:** Quinoa salad with salmon and roasted vegetables.

- **Dinner:** Lentil curry with turmeric, garlic, and kale.

- **Snack:** A few squares of 70% dark chocolate with a handful of berries.

Featured Recipes

Overnight Oats with Chia & Berries

- ½ cup rolled oats

- 1 cup unsweetened almond milk

- 1 tbsp chia seeds

- ½ cup blueberries

- 1 tsp cinnamon

Instructions: *Combine oats, chia seeds, and almond milk in a jar. Refrigerate overnight. In the morning, stir in cinnamon and top with blueberries.*

Turmeric Chicken Soup

- 2 chicken breasts, diced
- 1 onion, chopped
- 2 carrots, sliced
- 3 cups chicken broth
- 1 tsp turmeric
- 2 cups spinach

Instructions: *Sauté onion and carrots in olive oil, add chicken, turmeric, and broth. Simmer until chicken is cooked. Stir in spinach before serving.*

Salmon & Quinoa Bowl

- 1 salmon fillet

- ½ cup cooked quinoa

- 1 cup roasted vegetables (broccoli, zucchini, peppers)

- 1 tbsp olive oil

- Squeeze of lemon

Instructions: *Roast salmon at 400°F for 12–15 minutes. Serve over quinoa and roasted vegetables with olive oil and lemon.*

Reflections: What You'll Notice

As you complete this first week, pause to reflect. Many readers find:

- **Less bloating** after meals.

- **Reduced stiffness** in the mornings.

- **Steadier energy** throughout the day, without the usual afternoon crash.

- **Clearer focus** and a lighter mood.

You may not feel all of these changes immediately, but even small shifts are signs that your body is beginning to calm down and heal.

The Takeaway

Week 1 is all about simplicity: removing triggers and giving your body a taste of balance. The meals are straightforward, the flavors are nourishing, and the results are often surprisingly quick. By the end of this week, you'll already feel the difference—and you'll be ready to move into Week 2, where we'll focus on **healing your gut** for deeper, longer-lasting change.

Week 1 –
Calm the Fire

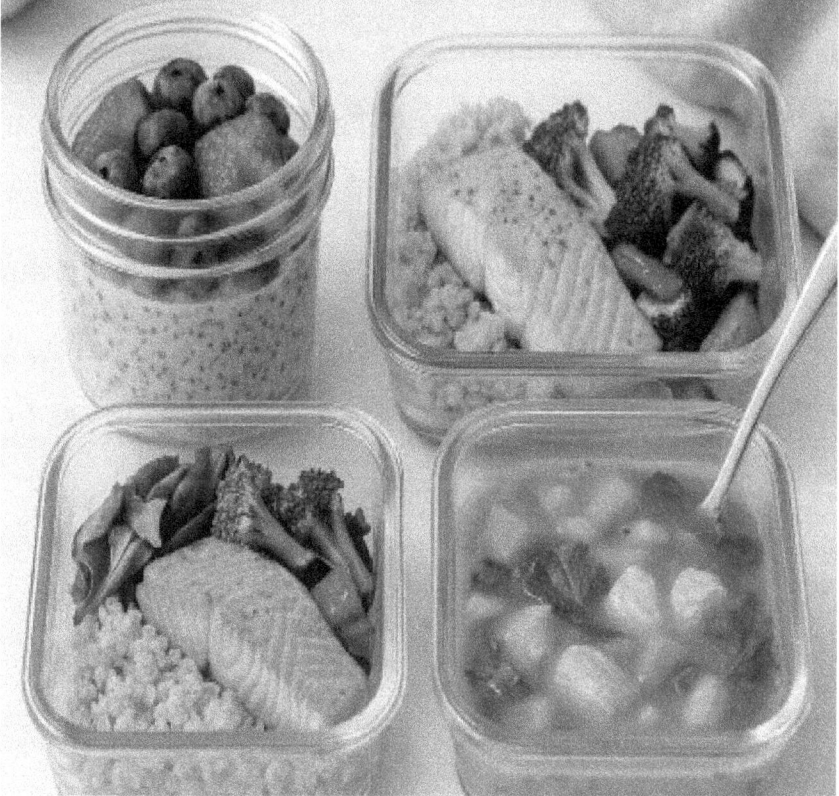

Chapter 5

Week 2 – Heal the Gut

By the time you finish your first week, the fire of inflammation has already begun to cool. You've removed the main triggers, and your body is starting to settle into balance. Now it's time to go deeper: to restore and strengthen one of the most important systems in your body—the gut.

Your digestive system is often called your "second brain" for good reason. It's home to trillions of microbes, collectively known as the gut microbiome. These tiny organisms influence everything from digestion to immunity, energy levels, and even mood. When the gut is balanced, you feel lighter, clearer, and more energized. When it's out of balance, inflammation takes root and spreads.

This week is all about feeding the good bacteria, improving digestion, and building diversity into your meals.

Focus: Adding Probiotics, Fiber, and Diversity

To heal your gut, three pillars matter most:

- **Probiotics:** These are live "good bacteria" that populate your gut, found in foods like yogurt, kefir, sauerkraut, miso, and kimchi.

- **Prebiotics:** These are the fibers and compounds in fruits, vegetables, and whole grains that feed probiotics and help them thrive.

- **Diversity:** The wider the variety of plants and whole foods you eat, the stronger and more resilient your microbiome becomes.

By combining these three, you create an internal environment where inflammation has less room to thrive.

Your 7-Day Plan

This week's meals focus on variety, flavor, and gut-friendly nourishment.

Day 1

- **Breakfast:** Greek yogurt parfait with blueberries, walnuts, and chia seeds.

- **Lunch:** Roasted veggie quinoa bowl with tahini dressing.

- **Dinner:** Miso soup with tofu, mushrooms, and spinach.

- Snack: Apple slices with almond butter.

Day 2

- **Breakfast:** Oatmeal topped with flaxseed, raspberries, and pumpkin seeds.

- **Lunch:** Lentil and chickpea salad with lemon-ginger dressing.

- **Dinner:** Grilled salmon with sautéed kale and garlic.

- **Snack:** A handful of walnuts and green tea.

Day 3

- **Breakfast:** Kefir smoothie with banana, spinach, and cinnamon.

- **Lunch:** Brown rice and roasted sweet potato bowl with avocado.

- **Dinner:** Turmeric chicken with broccoli and ginger-lime tea.

- **Snack:** Carrot sticks with hummus.

Day 4

- **Breakfast:** Chia seed pudding with almond milk and strawberries.

- **Lunch:** Quinoa tabbouleh with parsley, cucumber, and tomatoes.

- **Dinner:** Miso-glazed cod with bok choy and sesame seeds.

- **Snack:** A few squares of dark chocolate with blueberries.

Day 5

- **Breakfast:** Greek yogurt with ground flax and sliced peaches.

- **Lunch:** Roasted veggie and chickpea grain bowl with tahini.

- **Dinner:** Lentil curry with spinach and turmeric.

- **Snack:** Roasted almonds with ginger tea.

Day 6

- **Breakfast:** Kefir with chia seeds and raspberries.

- **Lunch:** Salmon avocado wraps in collard greens.

- **Dinner:** Miso soup with tofu, seaweed, and mushrooms.
- **Snack:** Cucumber slices with guacamole.

Day 7

- **Breakfast:** Overnight oats with pumpkin seeds, banana, and cinnamon.
- **Lunch:** Mediterranean lentil salad with olive oil and lemon.
- **Dinner:** Roasted chicken with garlic, sweet potato, and kale.
- **Snack:** Ginger-lime tea with a handful of walnuts.

Featured Recipes

Miso Soup with Tofu

- 3 cups vegetable broth
- 2 tbsp miso paste

- ½ cup tofu cubes

- 1 cup spinach

- ½ cup mushrooms, sliced

- 1 green onion, chopped

Instructions: *Warm broth, whisk in miso paste, then add tofu, mushrooms, and spinach. Simmer for 5 minutes. Garnish with green onion.*

Greek Yogurt Parfait

- 1 cup plain Greek yogurt

- ½ cup blueberries

- 1 tbsp walnuts, chopped

- 1 tbsp chia seeds

- Drizzle of honey (optional)

Instructions: *Layer yogurt with berries, nuts, and seeds in a glass or bowl. Chill for 10 minutes if desired.*

Roasted Veggie Quinoa Bowl

- 1 cup roasted vegetables (zucchini, peppers, carrots)
- ½ cup cooked quinoa
- 1 tbsp tahini
- Juice of ½ lemon

Instructions: *Toss roasted vegetables with quinoa, drizzle with tahini and lemon juice. Serve warm.*

Ginger-Lime Tea

- 1-inch fresh ginger root, sliced
- Juice of ½ lime
- 1 tsp honey (optional)
- 2 cups hot water

Instructions: *Steep ginger in hot water for 5 minutes. Stir in lime juice and honey. Serve warm.*

Reflections: What You'll Notice

As you finish Week 2, pause and notice what's shifting:

- **Better digestion:** less bloating, smoother bowel movements, more comfort after meals.

- **Clearer mind:** many experience reduced brain fog and steadier moods.

- **Fewer cravings:** with your gut nourished, sugar and processed food temptations often fade.

- **More energy:** balanced meals give you lasting fuel throughout the day.

Your gut is at the heart of your health, and this week you've given it exactly what it needs to begin healing.

The Takeaway

Healing your gut is one of the most powerful ways to fight chronic inflammation. By adding probiotics, prebiotics, and plant diversity, you're not just eating differently— you're rebuilding the foundation of your health.

In Week 3, you'll take everything you've learned and shift your focus toward boosting energy and creating lasting habits that will carry you beyond the reset.

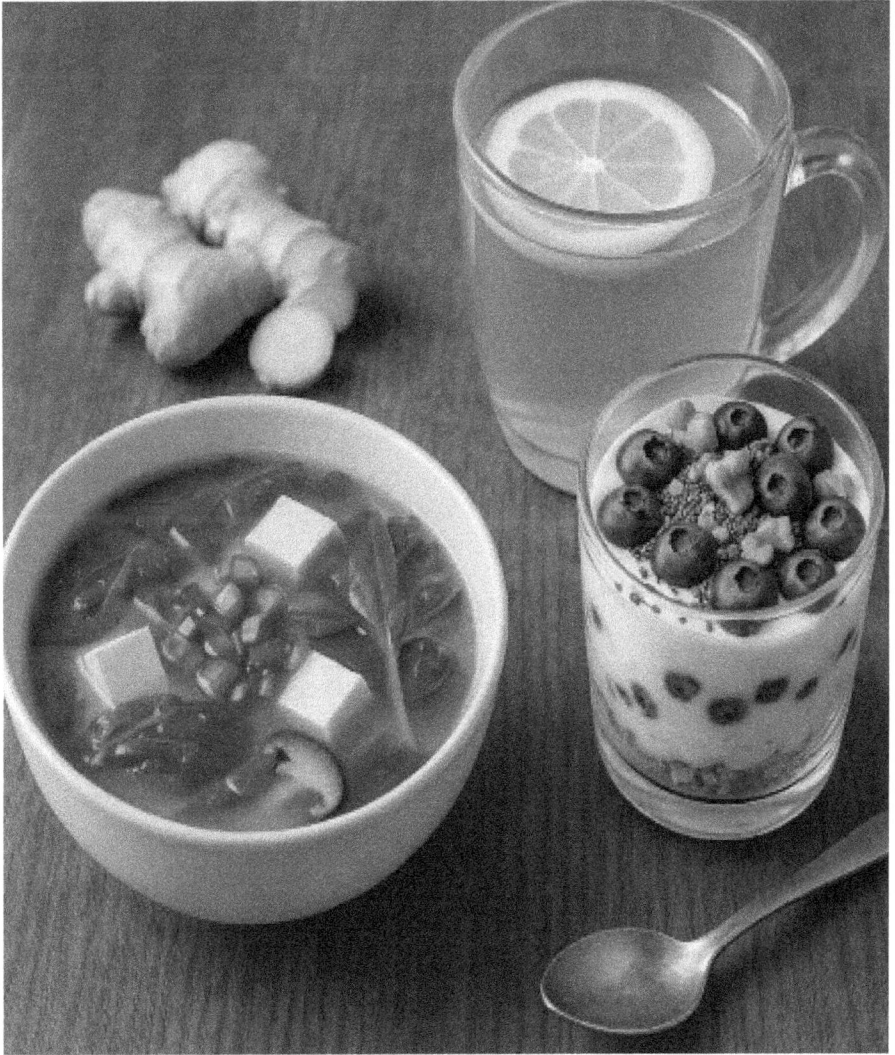

Chapter 6

Week 3 – Boost Energy & Build Lifelong Habits

By Week 3, your body has already experienced powerful changes: inflammation has calmed, digestion has improved, and you've started feeling lighter and more focused. This final week is about momentum—building on your progress to boost energy, sharpen focus, and establish habits that will carry you well beyond these 21 days.

This isn't about restriction anymore. It's about fueling your life with vibrant, energizing meals and creating a rhythm that feels natural, enjoyable, and sustainable.

Focus: Sustainable Anti-Inflammatory Living

Your body thrives when you give it steady nourishment and consistency. That's why this week emphasizes:

- **Energy-Boosting Foods:** Nutrient-dense meals with protein, complex carbs, and healthy fats to keep you fueled all day.

- **Meal Prepping Hacks:** Quick strategies to save time while eating well.

- **Lifestyle Habits:** Small daily choices—hydration, movement, rest—that anchor long-term success.

The goal is to leave this 21-day reset not just feeling better, but with the confidence that you can keep this going without feeling deprived or overwhelmed.

Your 7-Day Plan

Here's a sample plan for Week 3, filled with vibrant meals that energize both body and mind:

Day 1

71

- **Breakfast:** Green power smoothie (spinach, banana, almond butter, chia seeds).

- **Lunch:** Roasted veggie and quinoa bowl with tahini drizzle.

- **Dinner:** Shrimp stir-fry with broccoli, ginger, and garlic.

- **Snack:** Dark chocolate chia pudding.

Day 2

- **Breakfast:** Overnight oats with cinnamon, flax, and blueberries.

- **Lunch:** Lentil soup with turmeric and garlic.

- **Dinner:** Baked salmon with roasted sweet potatoes and spinach.

- **Snack:** Handful of walnuts and a green apple.

Day 3

- **Breakfast:** Scrambled eggs with spinach and avocado.

- **Lunch:** Mediterranean chickpea salad with olive oil and lemon.
- **Dinner:** Shrimp stir-fry with mixed vegetables and brown rice.
- **Snack:** Greek yogurt with raspberries.

Day 4

- **Breakfast:** Green power smoothie.
- **Lunch:** Roasted turkey lettuce wraps with avocado.
- **Dinner:** Turmeric lentil soup with kale.
- **Snack:** A few squares of dark chocolate with almonds.

Day 5

- **Breakfast:** Oatmeal with chia seeds, pumpkin seeds, and strawberries.
- **Lunch:** Quinoa tabbouleh with parsley, cucumber, and tomatoes.

- **Dinner:** Baked cod with lemon, garlic green beans, and wild rice.

- **Snack:** Ginger-lime tea with a handful of cashews.

Day 6

- **Breakfast:** Chia pudding with blueberries and walnuts.

- **Lunch:** Grilled chicken salad with mixed greens, olive oil, and avocado.

- **Dinner:** Shrimp stir-fry with zucchini noodles.

- **Snack:** A smoothie with kefir, banana, and spinach.

Day 7

- **Breakfast:** Green power smoothie.

- **Lunch:** Roasted vegetable and chickpea grain bowl.

- **Dinner:** Turmeric lentil soup with carrots and garlic flat-leaf parsley.

- **Snack:** Dark chocolate chia pudding.

Green Power Smoothie

- 2 cups spinach

- 1 banana

- 1 tbsp almond butter

- 1 tbsp chia seeds

- 1 cup unsweetened almond milk

Instructions: Blend all ingredients until smooth. Drink chilled.

Shrimp Stir-Fry

- 1 lb shrimp, peeled and deveined

- 2 cups broccoli florets

- 1 bell pepper, sliced

- 2 cloves garlic, minced

- 1 tbsp fresh ginger, grated
- 2 tbsp olive oil

Instructions: *Heat olive oil, sauté garlic and ginger. Add shrimp and vegetables, stir-fry until shrimp is pink and veggies are tender-crisp. Serve with brown rice or zucchini noodles.*

Turmeric Lentil Soup

- 1 cup red lentils, rinsed
- 1 onion, chopped
- 2 carrots, diced
- 3 cloves garlic, minced
- 1 tsp turmeric
- 4 cups vegetable broth

Instructions: *Sauté onion, carrots, and garlic in olive oil. Add lentils, turmeric, and broth. Simmer until lentils are soft. Blend slightly for creamier texture.*

Dark Chocolate Chia Pudding

- 3 tbsp chia seeds

- 1 cup almond milk

- 1 tbsp unsweetened cocoa powder

- 1 tsp honey (optional)

- A few squares of 70% dark chocolate, shaved for topping

Instructions: Mix chia seeds, almond milk, cocoa powder, and honey. Refrigerate overnight. Top with dark chocolate shavings before serving.

Reflections: Long-Term Rhythm

By now, you may be noticing:

- **More stable energy** throughout the day, with fewer slumps.

- **Better mental clarity**, as brain fog fades.

- **Easier meal choices**, since prepping and balance feel more natural.

- **Confidence in sustaining change**, because you've proven to yourself it's doable.

Take a moment each evening this week to reflect on what feels easier now compared to Day 1. That's proof of your transformation.

Meal Prepping Hacks for Busy Days

1. **Cook Once, Eat Twice:** Make extra portions at dinner and enjoy them for lunch the next day.

2. **Batch Cook Grains:** Prepare quinoa or rice at the start of the week for quick bowls.

3. **Pre-Chop Veggies:** Keep containers of chopped carrots, peppers, and greens in the fridge.

4. **Portable Snacks:** Portion out nuts, seeds, or chia pudding for grab-and-go energy.

Small habits like these save time, money, and energy—while keeping your anti-inflammatory lifestyle sustainable.

The Takeaway

Week 3 is where everything comes together. You're no longer just following a plan—you're living it. With energized mornings, steady afternoons, and satisfying meals, you've proven that anti-inflammatory living isn't a short-term reset, but a lifestyle you can enjoy long after these 21 days are done.

In the next part, you'll find the complete recipe collection, so you'll never run out of ideas to keep your meals diverse, flavorful, and healing.

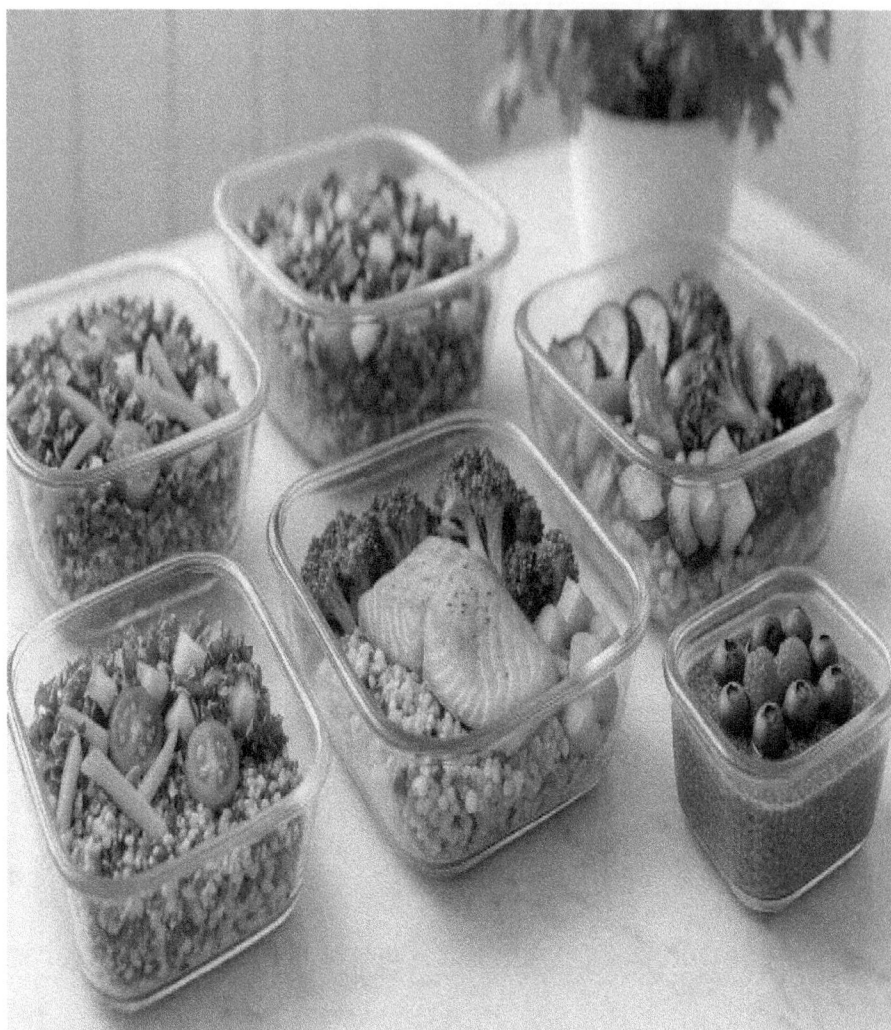

PART III – ANTI-INFLAMMATORY RECIPE COLLECTION (100+ RECIPES)

Chapter 7

Energizing Breakfasts

They say breakfast sets the tone for the day—and when it comes to anti-inflammatory living, that couldn't be more true. The first meal you eat either fuels your energy and focus or sets you up for crashes and cravings. This chapter is about creating **energizing breakfasts** that are quick, satisfying, and healing.

No matter your preference—savory or sweet, light or hearty—you'll find an option here. From eggs cooked with vibrant vegetables, to smoothies packed with greens and seeds, to hearty high-fiber bowls topped with fruit, every recipe is designed to keep inflammation low while boosting sustained energy.

Egg-Based Breakfasts: Protein to

Power Your Morning

Eggs are a near-perfect breakfast food: packed with protein, vitamins, and healthy fats. Pair them with vegetables and herbs, and you've got an anti-inflammatory powerhouse.

Spinach & Avocado Scramble

- 2 eggs
- 1 cup spinach
- ½ avocado, sliced
- 1 tsp olive oil
- Pinch of turmeric & black pepper

Instructions: Sauté spinach in olive oil, add whisked eggs, cook until soft. Top with avocado and turmeric.

Swap: Use scrambled tofu instead of eggs for a plant-based option.

Vegetable Omelet with Herbs

- 2 eggs or ½ cup egg whites
- ¼ cup chopped onions
- ¼ cup bell peppers
- Fresh parsley and basil

Instructions: Cook vegetables until tender, add whisked eggs, fold, and top with fresh herbs.

Swap: Use chickpea flour batter for a gluten-free vegan "omelet."

Smoothie-Based Breakfasts: Quick and Nutrient-Packed

Smoothies are perfect for busy mornings, and when balanced correctly, they provide long-lasting energy instead of sugar spikes.

Green Power Smoothie

- 2 cups spinach
- 1 banana
- 1 tbsp chia seeds
- 1 tbsp almond butter
- 1 cup almond milk

Instructions: *Blend until smooth.*

Swap: *Replace almond milk with coconut milk for a creamier, dairy-free variation.*

Berry Antioxidant Smoothie

- 1 cup mixed berries (blueberries, raspberries, strawberries)
- ½ cup Greek yogurt or coconut yogurt
- 1 tbsp flaxseed
- 1 cup water or almond milk

Instructions: *Blend until creamy.*

Swap: *Replace yogurt with silken tofu for a dairy-free protein boost.*

High-Fiber Bowls: Slow, Sustained Energy

Fiber is your friend when it comes to gut health and satiety. High-fiber bowls give you steady fuel throughout the morning and reduce mid-day crashes.

Overnight Oats with Chia & Berries

- ½ cup rolled oats (gluten-free if needed)
- 1 cup almond milk
- 1 tbsp chia seeds
- ½ cup blueberries
- Sprinkle of cinnamon

Instructions: Combine oats, chia, and milk in a jar. Refrigerate overnight. Add berries and cinnamon in the morning.

Quinoa Breakfast Bowl with Almonds & Apple

- ½ cup cooked quinoa
- ½ apple, sliced
- 1 tbsp almonds, chopped
- 1 tsp cinnamon
- Drizzle of honey (optional)

Instructions: *Warm quinoa, top with apple, almonds, and cinnamon.*

Swap: *Replace honey with dates or maple syrup if preferred.*

Chia Seed Pudding with Cacao

- 3 tbsp chia seeds
- 1 cup almond milk
- 1 tsp cacao powder
- 1 tsp vanilla extract

- Topped with strawberries

Instructions: *Stir chia, milk, cacao, and vanilla. Chill overnight until pudding-like.*

Swap: *Use coconut milk for a creamier, dairy-free option.*

Dairy-Free & Gluten-Free Swaps

- **Dairy-Free Yogurt Options:** Coconut, almond, or cashew yogurt.
- **Milk Alternatives:** Almond, oat, coconut, hemp, or soy milk.
- **Grain Alternatives:** Use gluten-free oats, quinoa, or buckwheat for bowls.
- **Protein Alternatives:** Tofu scrambles instead of eggs; silken tofu or pea protein in smoothies.

Reflections: How You'll Feel

By consistently starting your day with these breakfasts, you'll notice:

- Steady energy instead of sugar crashes.
- Sharper focus in the mornings.
- Reduced cravings mid-morning, since your meals are fiber- and protein-rich.
- Improved digestion thanks to probiotics, fiber, and nutrient-dense ingredients.

The Takeaway

Breakfast doesn't have to be complicated—it just has to be intentional. By leaning on eggs, smoothies, and high-fiber bowls, and using simple swaps for dairy and gluten, you'll start each day with power, clarity, and stability.

In the next chapter, we'll shift to **healing lunches** that travel well and keep you satisfied through the busiest part of your day.

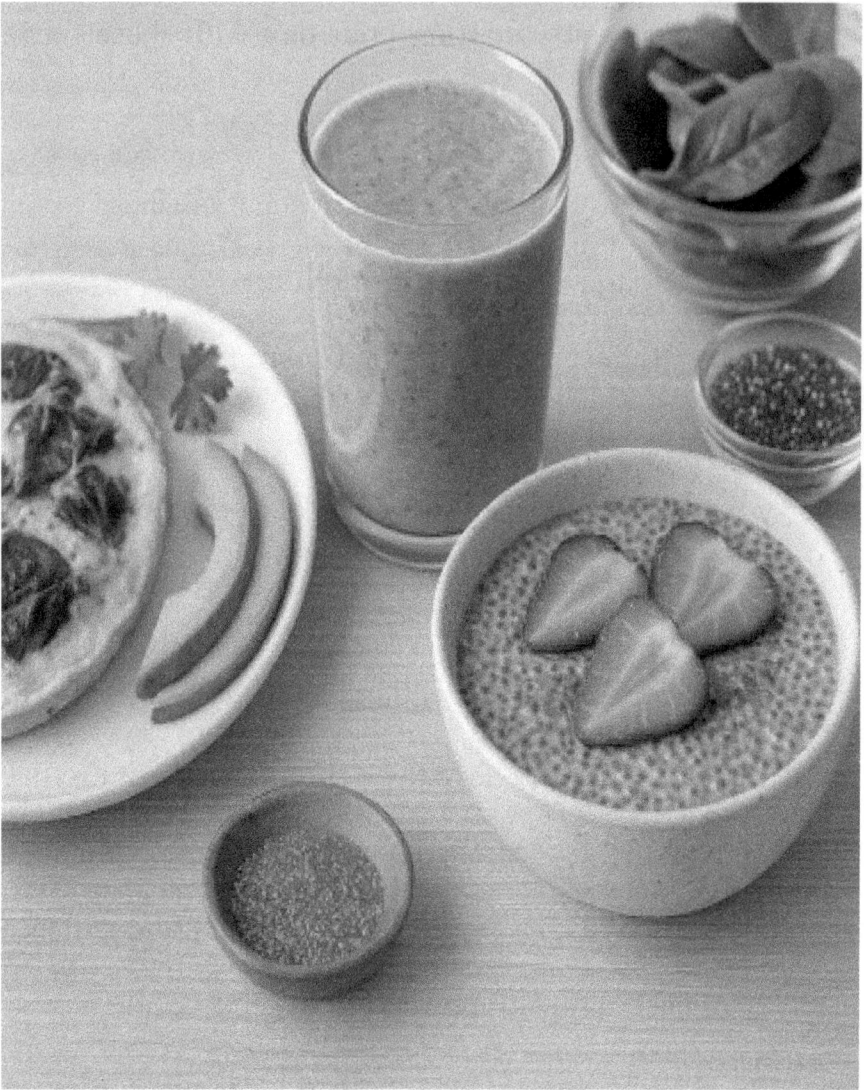

Chapter 8

Healing Lunches

Lunch is the meal that often gets neglected. It's easy to grab a quick sandwich, reheat leftovers, or skip it altogether during a busy day. But when you're living an anti-inflammatory lifestyle, lunch becomes one of your best opportunities to nourish your body, steady your energy, and prevent the dreaded afternoon slump.

The key is to make lunch both **healing and convenient—** meals that travel well, taste great, and keep you full for hours. This chapter focuses on **mason jar salads, hearty grain bowls, lettuce wraps, and thermos-friendly soups and stews**. These meals are colorful, nutrient-dense, and designed to fit into even the busiest schedule.

Mason Jar Salads: Layered,

Portable Healing

Mason jar salads are perfect for meal prep. By layering ingredients properly, you keep greens crisp and flavors fresh until lunchtime.

Mediterranean Mason Jar Salad

- Bottom: Lemon-olive oil vinaigrette
- Layer: Chickpeas, cucumber, cherry tomatoes
- Layer: Quinoa and parsley
- Top: Spinach and arugula

Instructions: Layer in order, keeping the dressing at the bottom and greens at the top. Shake before eating.

Swap: Replace chickpeas with grilled chicken or lentils for variety.

Rainbow Anti-Inflammatory Salad

- Bottom: Turmeric-tahini dressing

- Layer: Shredded carrots and red cabbage

- Layer: Roasted sweet potatoes

- Top: Kale and spinach

Instructions: *Store upright, shake well before serving.*

Tip: *Add pumpkin seeds for crunch and extra magnesium.*

Grain Bowls: Balanced Fuel in One Dish

Grain bowls offer flexibility and balance—protein, healthy fats, and fiber all in one bowl.

Quinoa & Roasted Veggie Bowl

- ½ cup cooked quinoa

- Roasted zucchini, broccoli, and peppers

- 1 tbsp tahini dressing

- ½ avocado, sliced

Instructions: *Assemble in a bowl or container. Drizzle with tahini before eating.*

Salmon & Brown Rice Bowl

- ½ cup cooked brown rice
- 1 grilled salmon fillet
- Steamed spinach and carrots
- Sprinkle of sesame seeds

Instructions: *Pack in a reheatable container. Enjoy warm or room temperature.*

Lettuce Wraps: Light and Satisfying

Lettuce wraps are an excellent way to enjoy healing proteins and vegetables without heavy carbs.

Turkey Avocado Lettuce Wraps

- Romaine or collard leaves

- Sliced turkey breast

- Avocado slices

- Shredded carrots and cucumbers

- Drizzle of olive oil and lemon

Instructions: Roll and secure with parchment paper for easy travel.

Chickpea & Veggie Wraps

- Romaine leaves

- Mashed chickpeas with olive oil and lemon

- Chopped red peppers and spinach

- Sprinkle of turmeric

Instructions: Fill leaves, roll gently, and pack tightly for travel.

Thermos-Friendly Soups & Stews

Soups and stews are comforting, easy to prepare in

batches, and perfect for carrying in a thermos to stay warm until lunch.

Turmeric Lentil Stew

- 1 cup red lentils, rinsed
- 1 onion, chopped
- 2 carrots, diced
- 1 tsp turmeric
- 4 cups vegetable broth

Instructions: Simmer all ingredients until lentils are tender. Portion into thermos containers.

Miso Veggie Soup

- 3 cups broth
- 2 tbsp miso paste
- Tofu cubes, spinach, and mushrooms
- Ginger slices

Instructions: Add miso paste to hot broth, stir in

vegetables and tofu. Keeps warm in a thermos.

Reflections: How Healing Lunches Feel

By upgrading your lunches, you'll notice:

- **Steadier energy** through the afternoon.

- **No more heavy post-lunch slump**, since these meals are balanced and light.

- **Improved digestion** thanks to fiber-rich veggies and gut-friendly ingredients.

- **Less snacking later**, because balanced lunches keep cravings in check.

The Takeaway

Lunch doesn't have to be a rushed sandwich or fast-food stop. With mason jar salads, grain bowls, lettuce wraps, and warming soups, you can create meals that heal your gut, steady your energy, and fit into any schedule.

In the next chapter, we'll shift to anti-inflammatory dinners—the comforting meals that wind down your day and continue the healing process into the evening.

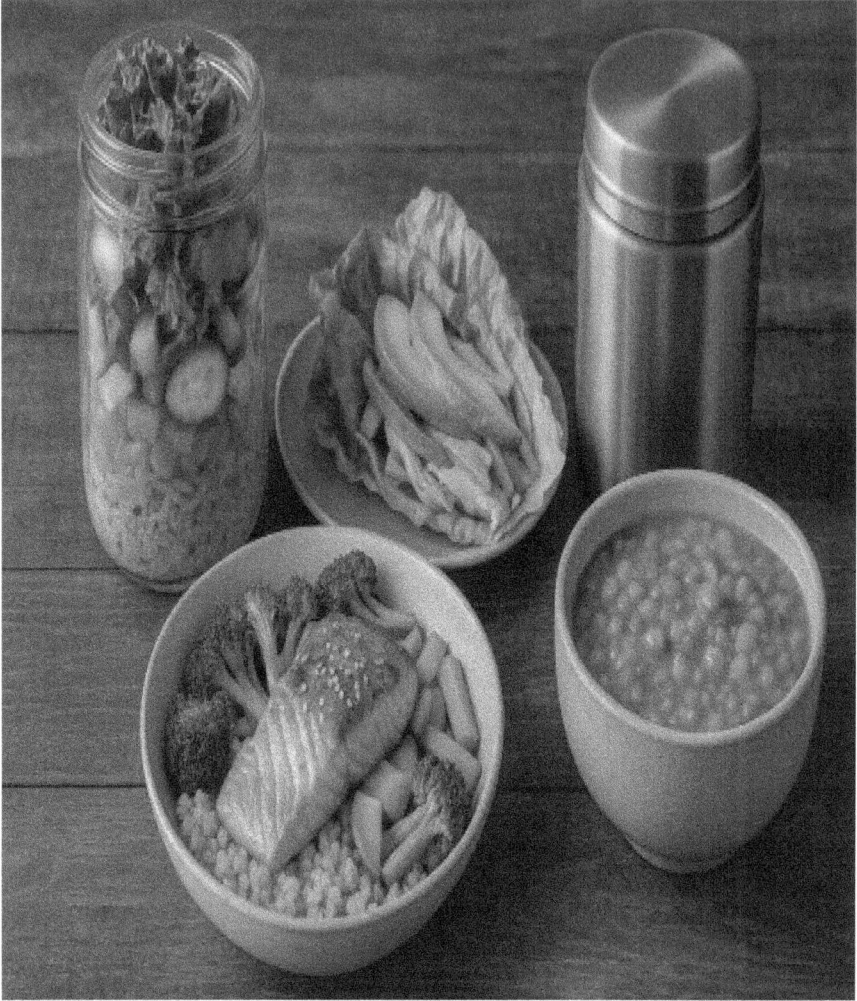

Chapter 9

Anti-Inflammatory Dinners

Dinner is where everything comes together. It's the meal that ends your day, nourishes your body overnight, and often becomes the center of family time. But it's also the meal where many people fall into the trap of takeout, heavy portions, or convenience foods that trigger inflammation.

This chapter shows you that anti-inflammatory dinners can be **easy, comforting, and deeply satisfying**. With one-pan meals, sheet-pan salmon, quick veggie stir-fries, and gut-friendly curries, you'll have options that save time without sacrificing flavor.

One-Pan Meals: Simple, Healing,

and Hassle-Free

Cooking on a single pan or skillet reduces stress and cleanup while locking in nutrients.

One-Pan Lemon Garlic Chicken with Veggies

- 2 chicken breasts
- 1 zucchini, sliced
- 1 cup broccoli florets
- 1 bell pepper, sliced
- Juice of 1 lemon
- 2 cloves garlic, minced
- 2 tbsp olive oil

Instructions: *Arrange chicken and vegetables on a skillet or baking dish. Drizzle with olive oil, lemon, and garlic. Bake at 400°F for 25 minutes.*

One-Pan Turmeric Shrimp & Quinoa

- 1 lb shrimp, peeled

- 1 cup cooked quinoa

- 1 cup spinach

- 1 tsp turmeric

- 1 tbsp olive oil

Instructions: *Heat oil in a skillet, sauté shrimp with turmeric until pink. Stir in spinach and quinoa. Serve warm.*

Sheet-Pan Salmon: Effortless & Flavorful

Sheet-pan dinners are a favorite for anti-inflammatory cooking—they're quick, nutrient-dense, and taste amazing.

Sheet-Pan Salmon with Broccoli & Sweet Potatoes

- 2 salmon fillets

- 1 cup broccoli florets

- 1 sweet potato, diced

- 1 tbsp olive oil

- 1 tsp paprika

- Sea salt & black pepper

Instructions: *Toss broccoli and sweet potatoes with oil and paprika. Spread on a sheet pan. Bake at 400°F for 15 minutes, then add salmon fillets and cook another 12 minutes.*

Herb-Crusted Salmon with Asparagus

- 2 salmon fillets

- 1 bunch asparagus

- 2 tbsp olive oil

- Fresh dill, parsley, lemon zest

***Instructions:** Place salmon and asparagus on a sheet pan, brush with olive oil, sprinkle with herbs and zest. Bake at 375°F for 15–18 minutes.*

Veggie Stir-Fries: Fast, Colorful, and Nutrient-Dense

Stir-fries are perfect for busy nights—just toss vegetables, protein, and spices into a wok for a healing, flavorful dinner in minutes.

Ginger-Garlic Veggie Stir-Fry

- 1 cup broccoli florets
- 1 red bell pepper
- 1 carrot, sliced
- ½ cup snap peas
- 2 cloves garlic, minced
- 1 tsp fresh ginger, grated

- 2 tbsp olive oil or avocado oil

Instructions: Heat oil in a wok. Add garlic and ginger, then vegetables. Stir-fry for 5–7 minutes until tender-crisp. Serve with quinoa or brown rice.

Tofu & Bok Choy Stir-Fry

- 1 block firm tofu, cubed

- 1 bunch bok choy

- 1 tbsp sesame seeds

- 1 tbsp tamari or coconut aminos

- 1 tsp ginger

Instructions: Pan-fry tofu until golden. Add bok choy and ginger. Drizzle with tamari and sprinkle with sesame seeds.

Gut-Friendly Curries: Comfort in a

Bowl

Curries are warming, deeply flavorful, and naturally anti-inflammatory when made with spices like turmeric, cumin, and ginger.

Golden Turmeric Lentil Curry

- 1 cup red lentils
- 1 onion, chopped
- 2 carrots, diced
- 1 tsp turmeric
- 1 tsp cumin
- 3 cups vegetable broth
- 1 cup coconut milk

Instructions: Sauté onion and carrots, add lentils, spices, and broth. Simmer until lentils are soft. Stir in coconut milk before serving.

Coconut Chickpea Curry

- 1 can chickpeas

- 1 zucchini, diced

- 1 red bell pepper

- 1 tsp curry powder

- 1 tsp turmeric

- 1 cup coconut milk

Instructions: *Sauté vegetables with spices, add chickpeas and coconut milk. Simmer for 15 minutes. Serve over brown rice.*

Reflections: How Anti-Inflammatory Dinners Change Your Evenings

As you embrace these dinners, you'll begin to notice:

- **Less heaviness at night**, because meals are nutrient-dense, not greasy.

106

- **Improved digestion** before bed, reducing bloating and discomfort.

- **Steadier energy into the evening**, without post-dinner fatigue.

- **More joy in cooking**, since these recipes are quick, colorful, and satisfying.

The Takeaway

Dinner should restore you, not drain you. By using simple one-pan meals, sheet-pan salmon, quick veggie stir-fries, and comforting gut-friendly curries, you're fueling your body with healing ingredients while keeping cooking stress-free.

With these dinners, you'll end each day feeling nourished, satisfied, and ready to carry your anti-inflammatory lifestyle into tomorrow.

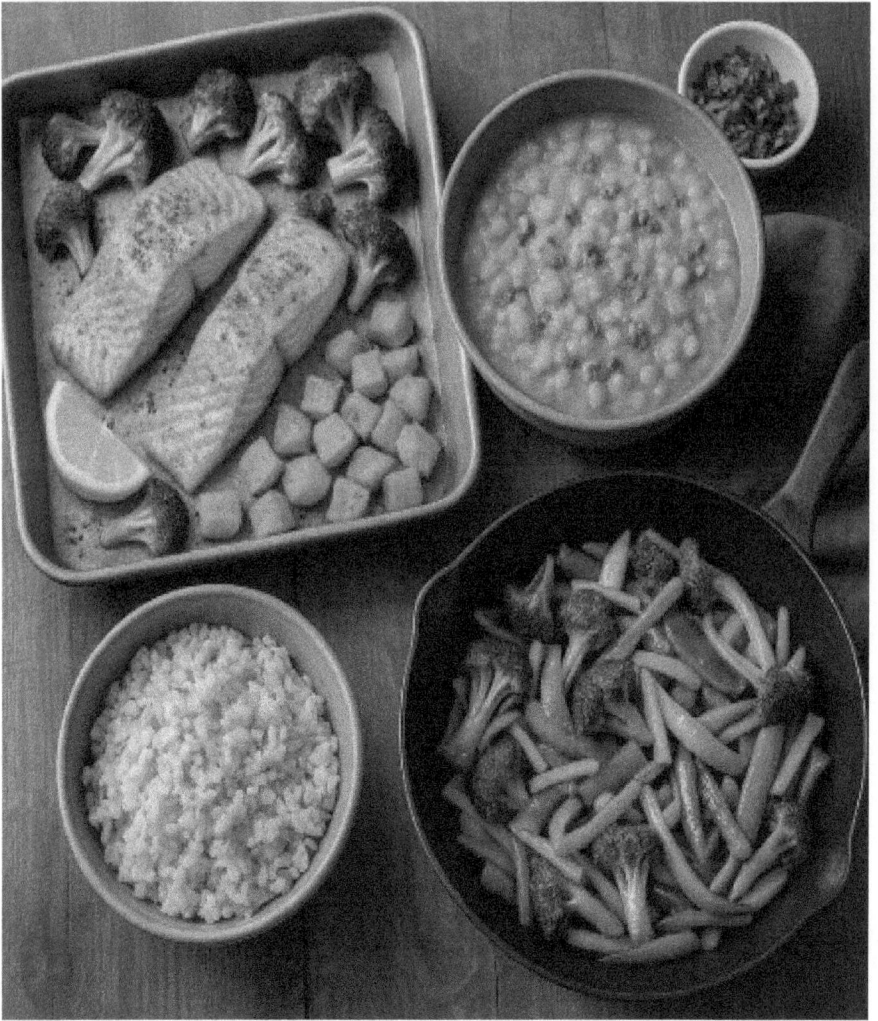

Chapter 10

Snacks & Small Bites

Snacks are often where healthy eating unravels. It's easy to grab a bag of chips, a candy bar, or a sugary drink when hunger hits between meals. But snacks don't have to be guilty pleasures—they can be powerful, healing small bites that keep inflammation low, cravings in check, and energy steady.

This chapter focuses on protein-rich dips, roasted nuts, and homemade bars—all easy to prepare, portable, and satisfying. With these options at hand, you'll no longer feel the need to reach for processed snacks.

Protein-Rich Dips

Classic Hummus with Turmeric Twist

- 1 can chickpeas, drained

- 2 tbsp tahini

- Juice of 1 lemon

- 1 clove garlic

- 1 tsp turmeric

- 2 tbsp olive oil

Instructions: *Blend all ingredients until smooth. Serve with cucumber sticks, carrot sticks, or celery.*

Greek Yogurt Herb Dip

- 1 cup plain Greek yogurt (or coconut yogurt for dairy-free)

- 1 tbsp olive oil

- Fresh dill, parsley, and mint, chopped

- 1 garlic clove, minced
- Pinch of sea salt

Instructions: Mix all ingredients. Chill for 30 minutes. Perfect for dipping raw veggies.

Guacamole with Flaxseed

- 2 ripe avocados
- Juice of 1 lime
- 1 small tomato, diced
- 1 tbsp ground flaxseed
- Sea salt & black pepper

Instructions: Mash avocados, stir in lime, tomato, and flaxseed. Enjoy with lettuce cups or veggie sticks.

Roasted Nuts

Rosemary Almonds

- 2 cups raw almonds
- 1 tbsp olive oil
- 1 tsp rosemary
- ½ tsp sea salt

Instructions: Toss almonds with oil and rosemary. Roast at 325°F for 15 minutes. Cool before storing.

Cinnamon Walnuts

- 2 cups raw walnuts
- 1 tsp cinnamon
- 1 tbsp maple syrup

Instructions: Mix walnuts with cinnamon and syrup. Bake at 300°F for 12 minutes. Great for an afternoon energy boost.

Spiced Pumpkin Seeds

- 1 cup pumpkin seeds
- 1 tsp paprika
- ½ tsp turmeric
- 1 tsp olive oil

Instructions: Toss seeds in oil and spices. Roast at 325°F for 10 minutes.

Homemade Bars

No-Bake Almond Energy Bars

- 1 cup rolled oats (gluten-free if needed)
- ½ cup almond butter
- ¼ cup honey or maple syrup
- ¼ cup chia seeds
- ½ cup chopped nuts

Instructions: Mix all ingredients. Press into a lined baking dish. Chill 2 hours, cut into bars.

Cacao Date Protein Bites

- 1 cup dates, pitted
- ½ cup almonds
- 2 tbsp cacao powder
- 1 tbsp chia seeds
- Pinch of sea salt

Instructions: Blend in a food processor until sticky. Roll into bite-sized balls. Refrigerate.

Coconut Cashew Bars

- 1 cup cashews
- ½ cup shredded coconut (unsweetened)
- ¼ cup coconut oil
- 1 tbsp honey

Instructions: Blend all ingredients, press into dish, chill until firm, cut into bars.

Reflections: How Snacks Can Heal

When your snacks are intentional, you'll notice:

- **No more sugar crashes**, since protein and healthy fats keep energy steady.

- **Less mindless snacking**, because these bites are truly satisfying.

- **Better digestion**, thanks to fiber, probiotics, and nutrient-dense ingredients.

- **More control**, since having prepared snacks on hand removes temptation.

The Takeaway

Snacks aren't the enemy—processed snacks are. By choosing dips, nuts, and homemade bars, you're fueling your body between meals with the same healing principles as your breakfasts, lunches, and dinners. These small bites may be quick, but their impact is long-lasting.

In the next chapter, we'll satisfy your sweet tooth with **guilt-free desserts** that comfort and heal at the same time.

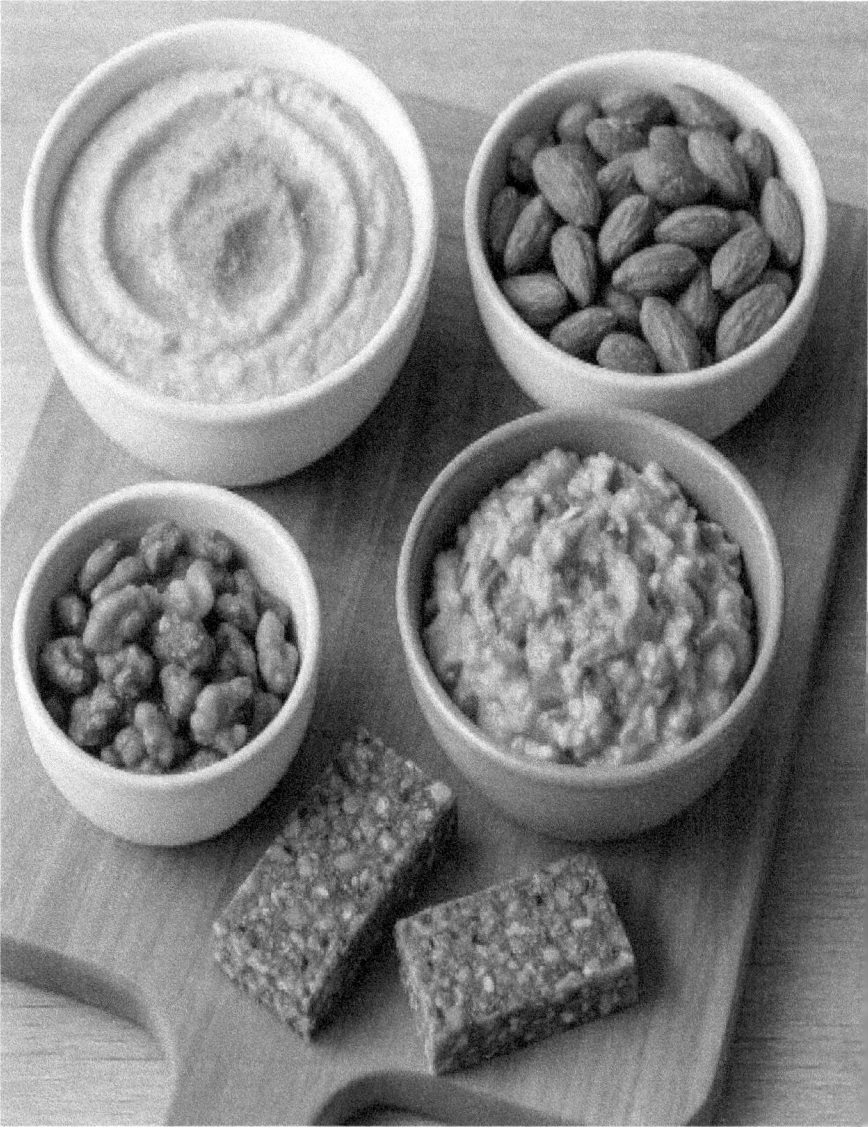

Chapter 11

Guilt-Free Desserts

For many people, dessert feels like the enemy of healthy eating—something to avoid, resist, or feel guilty about afterward. But in an anti-inflammatory lifestyle, desserts don't have to be off-limits. With the right ingredients, you can enjoy **sweet, satisfying treats** that actually nourish your body instead of harming it.

This chapter focuses on **chia puddings, fruit-based sweets, and dark chocolate energy bites**—easy-to-make desserts that bring joy, flavor, and healing in every bite. They're rich in fiber, healthy fats, and antioxidants, so you can indulge without the sugar crash.

Chia Puddings: Creamy, Satisfying,

and Healing

Chia seeds are tiny but powerful. Packed with fiber, omega-3 fatty acids, and protein, they create a pudding-like texture when soaked in liquid—making them the perfect base for guilt-free desserts.

Vanilla Berry Chia Pudding

- 3 tbsp chia seeds
- 1 cup almond milk
- 1 tsp vanilla extract
- 1 tsp honey or maple syrup
- ½ cup mixed berries

Instructions: Stir chia seeds, milk, vanilla, and honey. Refrigerate overnight. Top with berries before serving.

Chocolate Chia Delight

- 3 tbsp chia seeds

- 1 cup coconut milk
- 1 tbsp cacao powder
- 1 tsp honey (optional)
- Shaved dark chocolate

Instructions: Mix chia seeds, milk, and cacao. Chill overnight. Sprinkle with shaved dark chocolate before serving.

Golden Turmeric Chia Pudding

- 3 tbsp chia seeds
- 1 cup almond milk
- ½ tsp turmeric
- ¼ tsp cinnamon
- Pinch of black pepper
- 1 tsp maple syrup

Instructions: Combine ingredients, stir well, refrigerate overnight. The turmeric and cinnamon add warming, anti-inflammatory depth.

Fruit-Based Sweets: Nature's Candy

Fruit is naturally sweet and bursting with antioxidants. When paired with spices or light toppings, it becomes a dessert that satisfies cravings without refined sugar.

Honey-Roasted Pears

- 2 ripe pears, halved
- 1 tsp cinnamon
- 2 tsp honey
- Handful of walnuts

Instructions: Bake pears at 375°F for 20 minutes. Drizzle with honey, sprinkle cinnamon and walnuts.

Coconut Mango Parfait

- 1 cup coconut yogurt
- ½ cup fresh mango chunks
- 1 tbsp shredded coconut

- 1 tsp chia seeds

Instructions: *Layer yogurt, mango, coconut, and chia in a glass. Chill before serving.*

Baked Cinnamon Apples

- 2 apples, cored and sliced
- 1 tsp cinnamon
- 1 tbsp raisins
- 1 tsp maple syrup

Instructions: *Toss apples with cinnamon, raisins, and maple. Bake at 350°F for 15 minutes until tender.*

Dark Chocolate Energy Bites: Rich, Portable Treats

Dark chocolate (70% or higher) is loaded with antioxidants and magnesium, making it one of the best sweet indulgences in an anti-inflammatory lifestyle. Combined with nuts and seeds, it becomes both delicious and energizing.

Cacao Almond Energy Bites

- 1 cup almonds
- 1 cup dates, pitted
- 2 tbsp cacao powder
- 1 tbsp chia seeds
- Pinch of sea salt

Instructions: Blend in a food processor until sticky. Roll into balls. Refrigerate.

Coconut Chocolate Bliss Balls

- 1 cup shredded coconut
- ½ cup cashews
- 2 tbsp cacao powder
- 2 tbsp coconut oil

- 1 tbsp honey

Instructions: *Blend ingredients, roll into small balls, coat with extra coconut. Chill until firm.*

Dark Chocolate Pistachio Squares

- 1 cup dark chocolate, melted
- ½ cup pistachios, chopped
- 1 tbsp pumpkin seeds

Instructions: *Mix melted chocolate with nuts and seeds. Pour into a lined dish. Chill until hardened. Break into squares.*

Reflections: Sweet Without the Guilt

When you swap refined sugar and processed desserts for these nutrient-rich alternatives, you'll notice:

- **No more sugar crashes**, since fiber and protein balance the sweetness.

- **Sustained energy**, thanks to healthy fats and antioxidants.

- **Less guilt and more joy**, because dessert becomes part of your healing journey, not a setback.

- **Improved digestion**, since fruit, seeds, and nuts are easier on the gut than processed cakes or pastries.

The Takeaway

Dessert can be both indulgent and healing. With chia puddings, fruit-based sweets, and dark chocolate energy bites, you can enjoy sweet flavors while supporting your body's anti-inflammatory reset. These recipes prove that you don't need to give up pleasure—you just need to redefine it.

In the next chapter, we'll take your 21-day reset even further with a **full meal plan and grocery guide**, making it simple to keep this lifestyle going day after day.

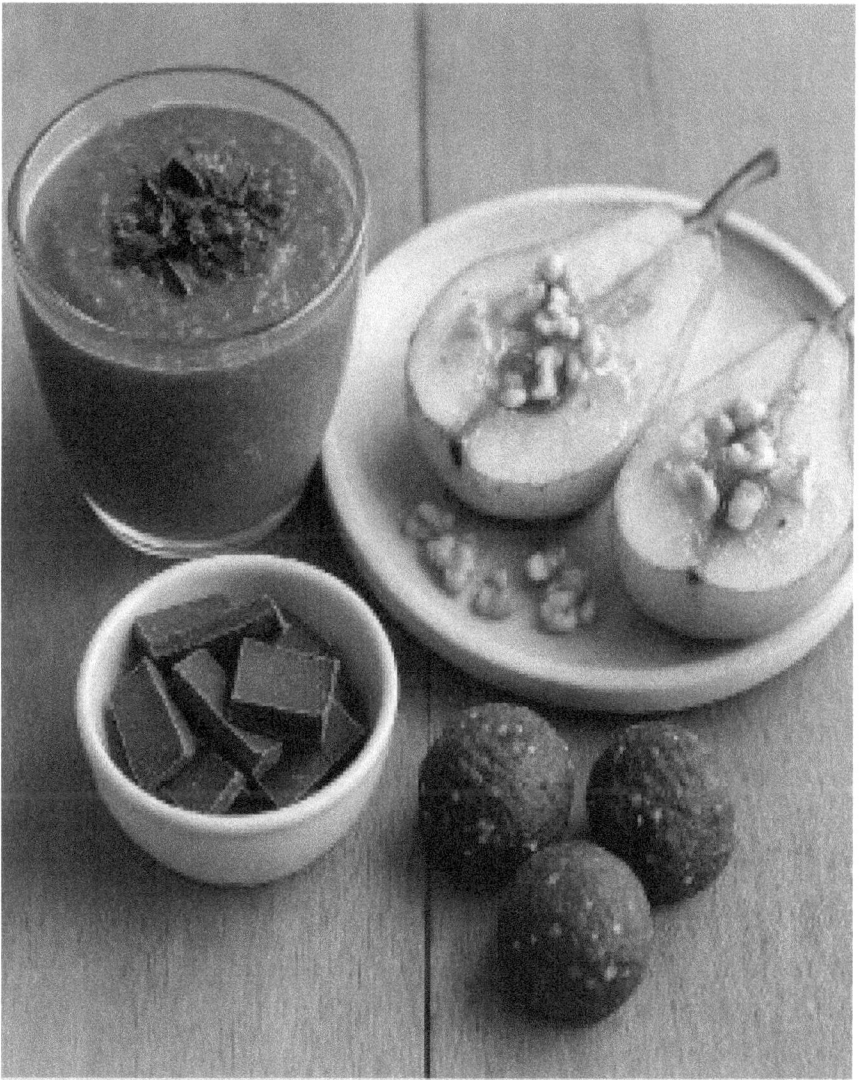

PART IV – LIVING THE LIFESTYLE

Chapter 12

Beyond 21 Days – Making It Stick

You've completed your 21-day reset. The fire has calmed, your gut is healing, and your energy feels renewed. But now comes the most important step: **making it stick**. The reset isn't the finish line—it's the foundation. The real transformation happens when anti-inflammatory living becomes your everyday rhythm, flexible enough to fit into real life but consistent enough to protect the progress you've made.

This chapter is about balance, resilience, and confidence. You'll learn how to navigate dining out, travel, holidays, and even slip-ups—without stress or guilt. Because true healing isn't about perfection; it's about building habits that can last a lifetime.

Dining Out Without Derailing Progress

One of the biggest fears after a reset is, "What happens when I eat out?" The good news is that restaurants can fit into your anti-inflammatory lifestyle if you make mindful choices.

Tips for Dining Out:

- **Scan the menu for whole foods.** Look for meals built around grilled fish, chicken, or legumes with vegetables and healthy fats.

- **Swap sides.** Replace fries or bread with steamed veggies, a side salad, or roasted potatoes.

- **Ask how it's cooked.** Request olive oil instead of butter, grilled instead of fried.

- **Watch the sauces.** Dressings and marinades often hide sugars or inflammatory oils. Ask for them on the side.

- **Enjoy mindfully.** Don't stress over small compromises. Focus on balance, not rigidity.

Travel Tips: Staying Balanced on the Road

Traveling can throw routines off, but with planning, it's possible to stay on track and feel good while away.

Smart Travel Strategies:

- **Pack snacks.** Bring roasted nuts, homemade bars, or fruit to avoid airport junk food.
- **Stay hydrated.** Carry a refillable water bottle and drink regularly to offset travel fatigue.
- **Choose wisely on the go.** Look for simple meals—grilled proteins, salads, grain bowls—rather than fast-food fried options.
- **Move daily.** Even 10 minutes of walking or stretching after long flights or drives helps reduce inflammation.

- **Relax the rules slightly.** Travel is about experience. Do your best, but don't let perfection steal the joy of the journey.

Celebrations Without Flare-Ups

Birthdays, holidays, weddings, and gatherings often revolve around food. Instead of dreading them, approach them with flexibility.

How to Celebrate Smart:

- **Bring a dish.** If you're unsure what will be served, contribute a salad, veggie platter, or anti-inflammatory dessert so you know there's a safe option.
- **Eat beforehand.** Have a small, balanced meal so you're not starving when faced with temptations.

- **Choose your indulgence.** Maybe it's a slice of cake or a glass of wine—but not both. Enjoy it slowly, guilt-free.

- **Focus on connection.** Celebrations are about people, not just food. Shift your attention to conversation, laughter, and memories.

Building Flexible Frameworks: The 80/20 Approach

Long-term success doesn't come from strict rules; it comes from flexibility. That's where the 80/20 approach shines.

- 80% of the time: Choose whole, anti-inflammatory foods—vegetables, fruits, lean proteins, whole grains, and healthy fats.

- 20% of the time: Allow room for life—occasional treats, dining out, or cultural foods you love.

This balance ensures you maintain progress without feeling restricted. It turns anti-inflammatory eating into a lifestyle instead of a diet.

How to Handle Slip-Ups Without Guilt

It's inevitable: there will be days when you eat the cake, grab the fries, or fall back into old habits. The difference now is how you respond.

Healthy Ways to Reset After a Slip-Up:

- **Don't spiral.** One meal doesn't undo weeks of progress.

- **Hydrate.** Drink water or lemon water to support digestion.

- **Rebalance your next meal.** Get back on track with a protein, leafy greens, and healthy fats.

- **Reflect, don't punish.** Ask yourself: Was it worth it? How did it make me feel? Use it as information, not guilt.

- **Keep perspective.** Progress is measured in consistency, not perfection.

The Takeaway

The real beauty of the anti-inflammatory lifestyle is its sustainability. You don't have to give up dining out, traveling, or celebrating life's joys. You don't have to fear slip-ups. With the right balance, mindfulness, and flexibility, you'll continue to feel lighter, more energized, and more in control.

This isn't just a 21-day reset anymore—it's your new way of living. And it's not about restriction; it's about freedom: the freedom to enjoy life without the constant weight of inflammation holding you back.

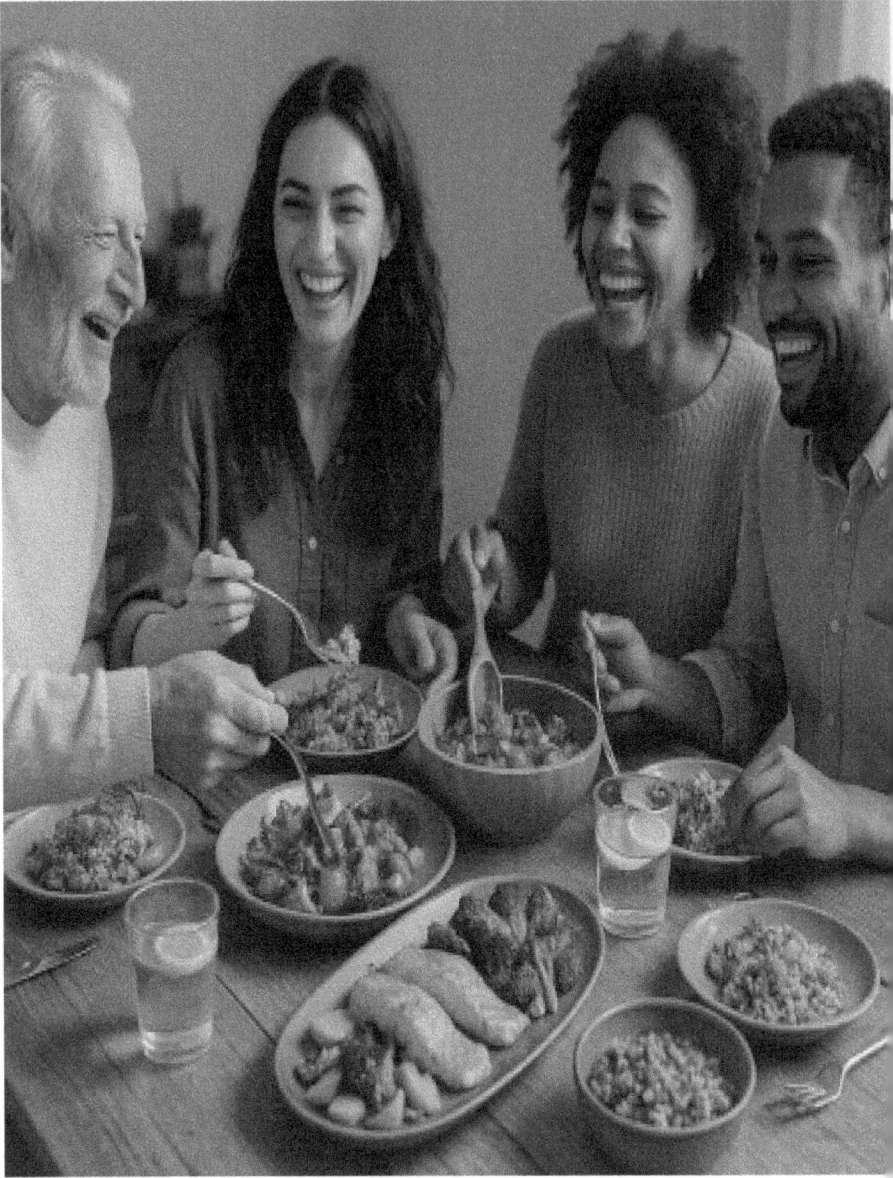

Glossary of Key Terms

Antioxidants: Natural compounds in fruits, vegetables, and dark chocolate that protect your cells from damage caused by free radicals.

Chronic Inflammation: Long-term, low-grade inflammation that lingers in the body and contributes to fatigue, joint pain, and chronic illness.

Free Radicals: Unstable molecules created by stress, pollution, or poor diet that can damage cells if not neutralized by antioxidants.

Omega-3 Fatty Acids: Healthy fats found in salmon, flaxseeds, and walnuts that reduce inflammation and support heart and brain health.

Phytonutrients: Plant-based compounds that help fight disease and support immune health; often found in colorful fruits and vegetables.

Probiotics: Live "good bacteria" that support digestion and balance the gut, found in yogurt, kefir, sauerkraut, and miso.

Prebiotics: Fibers in plant foods that feed probiotics, helping them thrive.

Turmeric: A golden spice containing curcumin, a powerful natural anti-inflammatory compound.

Acknowledgment

I wish to thank the countless individuals—readers, health practitioners, and nutrition experts—who have inspired this work. Your questions, insights, and shared experiences shaped this book into something practical and accessible. Above all, I am grateful to the community of everyday people seeking healthier, more energized lives; your determination proves that transformation is always possible.

www.ingramcontent.com/pod-product-compliance
Lightning Source LLC
Chambersburg PA
CBHW031128020426
42333CB00012B/284